HOW TO GET ABS

Contents

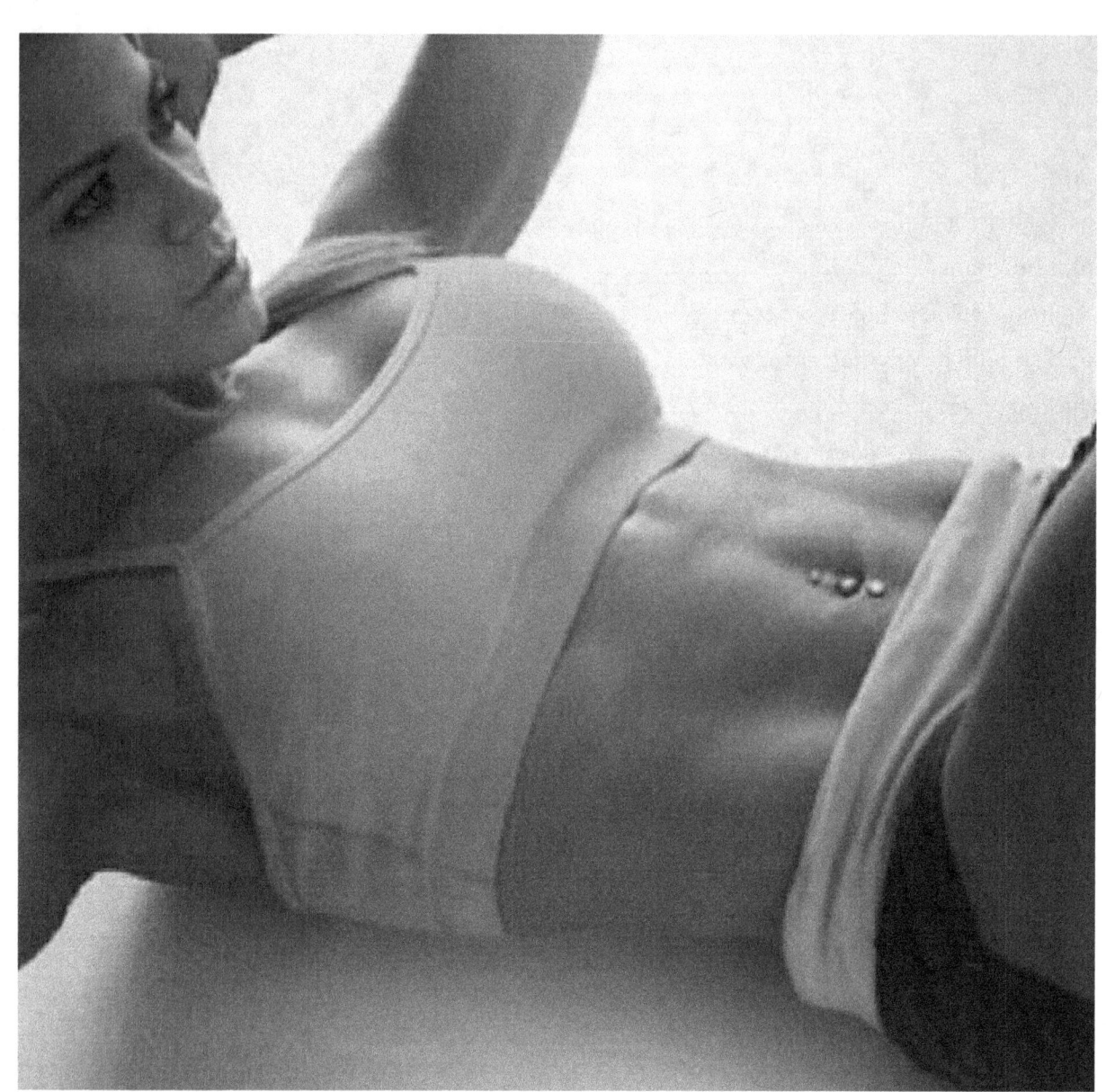

The flat ab dream

Getting a flat stomach is a dream for many. Reading about people getting it or looking at pictures in a magazine may make you wonder if you can create the same magic in your body. If you struggling with such notions, now is the time to let go of your inhibitions and start looking at how it can be done. We have listed some basic exercise moves and other mediums which will help you achieve your dream body.

Flat stomach exercises

Who doesn't want that very flattering flat abs look. Get into shape easy and fast with these easy and simple exercises? Also get firmer thighs and back while you are at it!

Pike and Extend

Lie down on the floor. Facing upwards, extend your legs over hips with arms extended overhead. Now crunch up trying to reach your feet.

Now keeping your legs straight, bring your arms overhead while lowering upper back and left leg towards the floor. Again crunch up, raising your left leg over your hips while trying to touch your toes. Repeat the same with opposite legs.

Side crunch while standing

Stand on left leg with left arm extended outwards at the height of the shoulder. Right foot should be lifted a few inches above the floor to the side. Place right hand behind your head with elbows bent out side wards at shoulder level. Then raise your right knee towards right elbow. Switch sides and repeat.

Chest fly with extended legs

Lie on the floor while facing upwards. Knees need to bend at 90 degrees over hips. Hold a dumbbell in each hand while your arms are extended over your chest while palms facing in wards. Keep right knee bent while straightening left leg toward the floor as you lower your arms towards the sides. Hold for a while and return to top. Switch legs and repeat.

Knee up with overhead press

Sit on the floor while bending your knees and feet firmly on the floor. Hold your dumbbells near the shoulder with elbows by your side and palms facing inwards. Lean backwards and stretch your arms overhead as you lift your feet a few inches above the floor while brining your knees towards the chest. Hold position and count to 3. Repeat about 15 times for best results.

Lunge and twist

Stand upright with feet together. Lunge backwards with your left leg while bending your knees at 90 degrees. Try to reach your right foot with your left hand. Stand up again and raise your left knee in front to the height of your hip. Bring your fists closer to your chest while bending elbows out to your sides as you twist to your left. Then twist back to center and lunge left leg back. Repeat the whole process and switch sides.

Clock exercise

Using an exercise ball, rest your back on it while your feet is aligned with your hips. Stretch arms over your head and contract your ab muscles. Start rotating your body like a clock. Carry out 10 rotations on each side.

Planks

Lie on the floor facing the downwards. Upper body should be supported on your forearms. Try lifting your entire body off the floor. Keep your toes in a straight line. Repeat thrice and then break for 15s.

Side work outs

Standing straight with your feet wide apart, approximately the width of your hips, slowly bend your knees while holding dumbbells in your both hands. Lift your hands above your head and relax. Lean towards your right and raise your arms, hold position and then relax. Repeat for left side.

Bicycle exercises

Lie on the floor and place your hands under your head and raise your knees off the floor. Bring right elbow towards the left knee while performing a cycling motion. Switch elbows and repeat

Dumbbell bends

Hold a dumbbell in your right hand in such a way that your palm is facing the body. Feet should be at a shoulder width distance and slowly place your left hand on your hip. Bend upper body to the right side while facing the front. Bring your body back to normal posture and repeat with the left side.

Perpendicular exercise

Lie on your back with your arms behind your back. Lift your legs over your hips at 90 degrees and breathe out. Then widen the gap between your legs. Breathe in as you lower your legs. Do a set of 5- 10 as you progress.

Funky standing abs

Stand straight in the beginning. Next bend your knees and tighten your abs gradually. Push your pelvis forward so your back is curved. Return to original position and repeat the same by tilting your pelvis in the backward direction. Repeat the same in either direction for 15 times.

Chair leg lifts

Sit straight with your back resting on the chair. Your back should be flat against the chair. Place your hands on the seat of the chair and slowly raise your knees towards your chest and put them back. Breathe slowly while performing this. Do a set of two and repeat 15 times.

Crunches

The basic crunches are also essential for any kind of ab workout routine. Lie flat on the ground with feet placed firmly on them and place your hand under your head. Lift just upper body and hold for about 3 seconds. Repeat a set of 15-20 and break. Step up the number of repeats as your progress. This is a complete exercise as it targets not only the mid-section area, but the upper abdomen, the lower abdomen and the oblique abdominal muscles as well.

Flat Ab belt

The abdominal muscles are the hardest of all to get under control during a weight loss program. An Ab belt may go a long way to help you reach that point where enviable abs are your assets. The belt is designed such that it can be used by anyone at any age. There are a variety of moves that you can try with the ab belt but we have mentioned the most effective and popular one here

The Rowboat routine- Sit on the floor, bend your knees a little and feet should hip width apart. Your heels should be firmly in place to provide balance to your body. Loop the belt around your feet and hold the handles in each hand. Your elbows should be by your side and bent at 90 degrees, while palms facing upwards. Keeping your core tight, lean torso backwards at 45 degrees and curl handle to shoulder. Hold position for 3 seconds and repeat a similar move by hinging to the front and stretching arms towards the sides, while keeping elbows close to your body. Do 16 repetitions of this entire exercise from the top.

Flat Ab Pills-

There are some flat ab pills also available in the market to help you further with attaining a flat stomach. It needs to be remembered that these pills don't aid in weight loss, they are essentially food supplements. However, it does accelerate the process through its laxative properties.

The ultimate goal is to build muscles and concentrate on burning fat. If you are able to reduce weight before you begin your muscle toning work outs, is equally beneficial as toning up your muscles before you start cutting down on body fat. All depends on how motivated you are towards your goal of achieving that perfectly toned body.

Besides the regular work out and diets, you must follow an active and healthy lifestyle. Full body exercises like running, skipping or swimming helps burn fat while elevating your heart rate. Nutritious intake is essential to control on the fat intake in the body. Understand the importance of good and bad fat. A balanced diet is essential for losing that belly fat. Also, drinking plenty of water and limiting salt intake will help fight off stress levels and reduce chances of putting on weight.

Please check out my book series "HOW TO GET ABS" and get in the best shape of your life:

http://www.amazon.com/dp/B00SSFWCPA

http://www.amazon.com/dp/B00QJJFS1C

http://www.amazon.com/dp/B00SX58DUI

Check out my other weight loss and Nutrition Books at:

http://www.amazon.com/dp/B00QH7DY4Y

http://www.amazon.com/dp/B00RVX3KY2

http://www.amazon.com/dp/B00QDHXN7Q

http://www.amazon.com/dp/B00PP8OZJ4

http://www.amazon.com/dp/B00PO0IQIO

You can get access my Free Weight Loss Video at www.achieveitforyou.com

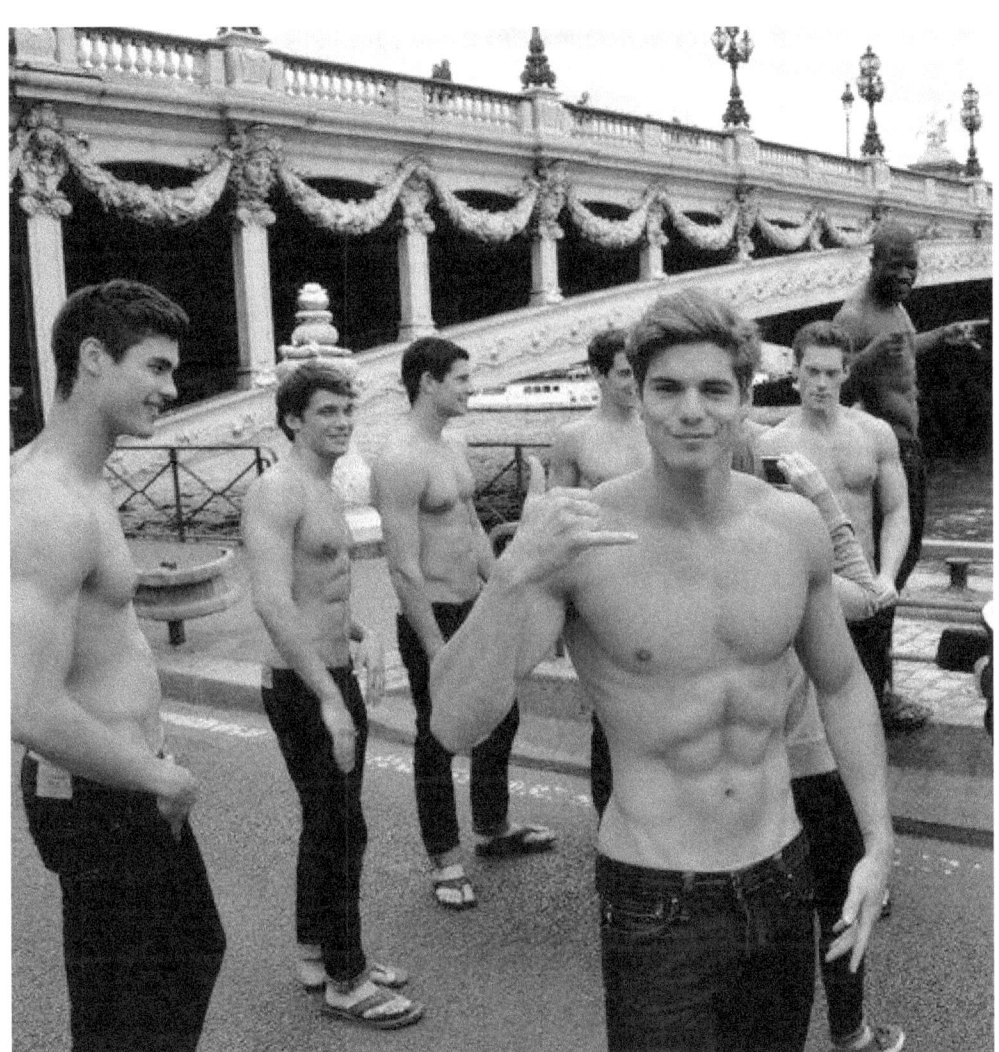

Fitness programs

Living your life with a perfectly sculpted body and a fit form isn't reserved for just professional trainers at the gym or serious athletes. Living a fit lifestyle is for everyone. A fit strong body is an asset that everyone should possess- grandparents, mothers, fathers, children and co employees. Whether you are training for a marathon or just a great body, fitness is essential. Training your mind and body to reach your fitness goals should be done through smart planning and some dedication. You should be able to cover all aspects like nutrition, motivation and training through your fitness programs to get to your goals.

Putting your body through a scheduled fitness program could be one of the best gifts that you present yourself. Physical exertion will reduce a risk of chronic heart disease, improve concentration power, help reduce weight, better your coordination, improves sleeping habits and your self-esteem. One should remember when launching yourself into an exercise regime, its essential to keep everything realistic. Careful planning and the right pace will establish a healthy lifestyle which will stay with you forever.

So if you intend to throw yourself into a strict regime and get your fitness a boost, follow these basic steps and you are good to go-

Measure your fitness level-

It is important to know where you stand so assessing your fitness is a good idea. You must already have a fair idea but scoring it will give you a better idea on how much you need to work on. You can create benchmarks and then assess your progress. Measuring your fitness level includes flexibility, body composition, muscular strength and aerobic fitness. You can make an informed judgment by recording the following-

- Pulse rate before and after you take a walk

- Duration of walk

- The point to which you can reach out to while sitting on the floor and trying to touch your toes

- Waist circumference, measured on top of your hip bone

- Your BMI count

Create your fitness program-

- Random exercise daily will not help your body. To optimize your efforts, a listed workout routine is required. You must work on a plan which is realistic and at the same time effective. Keep certain points in mind while designing a fitness program for yourself-

- What's your intent behind the program? Do you aim to lose weight, do you aim to put on weight? Are you just prepping for a marathon? Keeping your goals clear in your head will help you design the right plan

- Designing a balanced workout routine schedule is essential. A workout schedule ranging from 8 to 12 hours a week is ideal. This should include 75 minutes of intense aerobic activity. This should be combined with strength training also.

- Respect your pace. At the beginning remember to go slow and steady. If you get injured then see a doctor immediately and resume only after you have recovered fully. The program should up your stamina, endurance and strength gradually.

- Include an active lifestyle into your daily routine. In case you miss your cycling or treadmill, try and work your chores around them. Maybe catch your favorite soap while riding your stationary cycle.

- Mixing up your activities will maximize effectiveness and keep you from getting bored. This also minimizes the chances of an injury. Plan the exercises in such a manner that it targets different areas of the body.

- Resting after working out is important. Too much zeal can sometimes be a bad thing. Frenzied exercising will lead to sore muscles and aching joints.

- You can type out a list of what needs to done when and which day. You can create a time table with timings mentioned against the days. This will keep you on track and act as an additional motivator.

Assemble your fitness devices-

The basic thing to buy are good shoes. Ensure you buy the right kind again keeping your goal in mind. While buying the equipment, buy something which is easy to move around the house, easy to use and practical. You can also visit the fitness stores and get a trial use before buying. This will help you to make the right choice.

Start on your work out-

Once your gears or gym equipment's are in place and you are mentally prepped to get started, keep some tips handy to avoid the usual stumbles-

- Begin at a slow pace and spend a good amount of time in warming up. This can be done through some stretching exercises and general walking. Gradually increase your pace while making sure you rest if you over tire yourself while working out. The steady increase will add to your stamina and help you last longer during the work outs

- Break up your workout schedule. It's always a good idea to mix up your workout routine to prevent boredom and optimize effectiveness.

- Creativity should be your friend while mixing up your workout routine. Throw in other activities like jogging, swimming and cycling with your regular schedule. You can also join dance classes with your partner or go camping, trekking, or bike riding with your family.

- Be conscious of your body's needs. If you experience stress or pain while working out, take a break. Any kind of dizziness or shortness of breath is a poor sign and workouts should immediately be stopped.

- Be realistic with your goals. Don't push yourself so hard that you lose all motivation to continue. Try being easy on yourself at first.

Measure your progress-

Monitoring how much you have progressed is a big and important part of this regime. While fixing a schedule for yourself, fix a time period at regular intervals when you will gauge how much you have benefitted. This will help you assess how much more you need to put it to reach your goal or maybe ask you to slow down if you are progressing a little too fast.

Get a partner-

This may prove difficult to exercise as an option but try to rope in a friend, a family member or your partner. You can keep each other motivated and help reach your targets on time.

Please check out my book series "HOW TO GET ABS" and get in the best shape of your life:

http://www.amazon.com/dp/B00SSFWCPA

http://www.amazon.com/dp/B00QJJFS1C

http://www.amazon.com/dp/B00SX58DUI

Check out my other weight loss and Nutrition Books at:

http://www.amazon.com/dp/B00QH7DY4Y

http://www.amazon.com/dp/B00RVX3KY2

http://www.amazon.com/dp/B00QDHXN7Q

http://www.amazon.com/dp/B00PP8OZJ4

http://www.amazon.com/dp/B00PO0IQIO

You can get access my Free Weight Loss Video at www.achieveitforyou.com

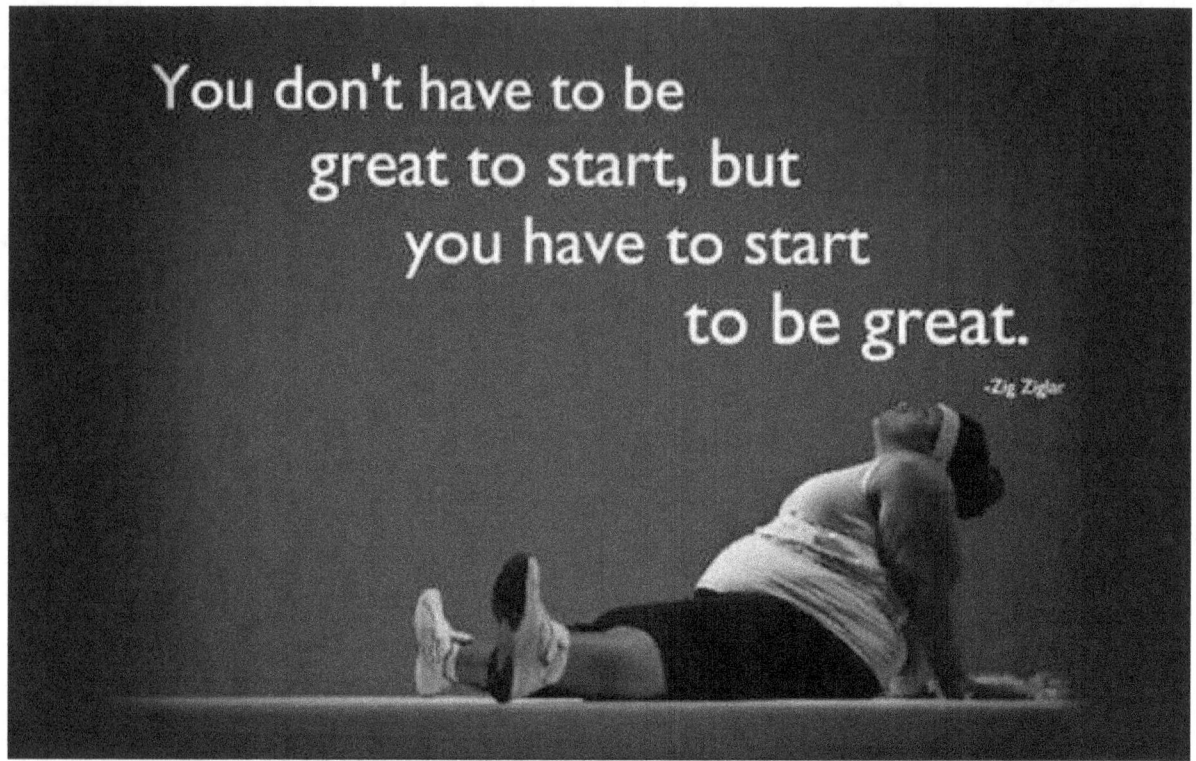

A beginner's guide to fitness programs

The first step is to you prepare yourself psychologically that you intend to get fitter and finer. Exercise can work like magic for your mind and body. Right from heart diseases to arthritis to helping people fight depression, exercise can be your magic wand. Of course there are the most common benefits to look forward to – weight loss and a well-toned body. It is important that you become consistent in your resolve to pursue a trimmed physique or a better heart. That of course doesn't mean you beat yourself up unfairly with a strict diet and an all-day at the gym session. The idea is to help get to a fitter body in a positive state of mind. Even a bit of physical activity everyday will give a boost to your overall well-being.

The exercise options are many like jogging, swimming and cycling. Even household related chores like gardening or dusting will help you keep you on your toes. It is essential you enjoy these activities as it will increase your chances of forming it into a habit.

The ideal amount of exercise daily, in case you are looking to lose weight is 30 minutes. This includes both walking/running and intense work out. It doesn't matter if you do less than 30 minutes per day, benefits will still show but not as quick.

When starting out, it's important to assess what kind of physical activity will suit you. This is directly correlated to your current fitness. If you are just a beginner, then intense aerobic work outs may cause you an injury, sabotaging all your hopes of a fitter body. If you are on the older side of 50, it's always recommended that you get a thorough medical check-up done before you commence on your mission. Share your work out plans with your doctor. He/she will guide you better. Medical issues may arise or present ones may worsen if we combine it with the wrong kind of exercise. Also set some goals. Do you want to participate in a sprinting competition or just lose weight, especially around your stomach? These goals should be crisp and clear in your head.

Do not become overly enthusiastic or aggressive right at the start. People dropping out because they don't see instant results is pretty common. Try to avoid falling into the trap and keep your determination alive. Aggressive workouts will also lead to injuries rather than producing the magical result. It's usually the over enthusiastic lot who drop out the fastest. So hang in there and see the expected results come in when it will matter the most. Try making a habit out of your regular regime so it doesn't look or feel tedious.

Beginner usually suffer from misconceptions about work out terms. They usually derive meanings from here say or make up their own ideas about them. Please follow the below list of terms and phrases you will come across when setting out to reach that desirable body-

Aerobics workout- This refers to the cardiovascular activity. These are strenuous exercises which will speed up your heart rate and breathing. Walking, sprinting, cycling and dancing may fall into this section

Max Heart beat rate- Refers to the maximum count that a person's heart beat can obtain. This is an age related number and can be obtained by subtracting your age from a total figure of 220.

Stretching- This is to get your muscles and joints into motion. If inactive, muscles and ligaments tend to shrink in size and keep reducing with time. A common misconception here is that stretching is equivalent to a warm up. What is true is that stretching is followed by a warm up session. If we try to stretch while our joints are cold, then it will lead to injuries.

Weight training- This kind of training is intended to improve strength of muscles in the body. This will involve lifting weights while focusing on different body area. You can lift weight with your arms and legs as per the instruction. This is also done with stretchy resistance bands to do push ups to work against your own bodyweight.

Sets- This is also a kind of strength training exercise. It involves repeating the same exercise for a particular number of times to form a set. For example you may do a set of 25 push ups or a set of 10 bicep curls

Reps- This again refers to the particular number of times you repeat the exercise.

Warm Up- Essential and the first thing you do when you begin working out. It's to prep your body for what is in store for next 30 odd minutes. This can be done with light aerobic work outs like slow walking. This helps increase the body temperature, increase blood flow and heating up joints and muscles. It's basically a lubricant for starting out. You can follow a warm up session with stretching exercises ideally.

The most important function of a warm up is it reduces chances of a muscle injury or prevents us from getting hurt.

Cooling down- This is the exact opposite to warm ups. This is to conclude the work out session by doing some light exercises. Some stretching followed by a few minutes' walk on the tread mill will bring down your heart rate and the body temperature to the normal level.

Gym equipment- Fitness can be achieved not only in gymnasiums but in the comforts of your home as well. With the right equipment and gears you can set up your very own gym at home. You can easily invest in the following gears and get started-

Treadmill- The most popular of all gym equipment perhaps. Try walking slowly for first 20 minutes and then speed up gradually to a slow jog. You can adjust the difficulty by playing with the incline level.

Ab exercise ball- The ab exercise ball may come with an instruction video or pamphlets. Follow the instructions well or you can check out videos online. Be careful not to slip and fall off. Once you get a hang of it, you will surely enjoy using it the most.

Weights- Dumbbells and Barbells are usually used to work on your strength building for the sides. Buy the weight that you can realistically work with and move up gradually.

You may additionally want to work in front of a mirror to get your form right as well.

Please check out my book series "HOW TO GET ABS" and get in the best shape of your life:

http://www.amazon.com/dp/B00SSFWCPA

http://www.amazon.com/dp/B00QJJFS1C

http://www.amazon.com/dp/B00SX58DUI

Check out my other weight loss and Nutrition Books at:

http://www.amazon.com/dp/B00QH7DY4Y

http://www.amazon.com/dp/B00RVX3KY2

http://www.amazon.com/dp/B00QDHXN7Q

http://www.amazon.com/dp/B00PP8OZJ4

http://www.amazon.com/dp/B00PO0IQIO

You can get access my Free Weight Loss Video at www.achieveitforyou.com

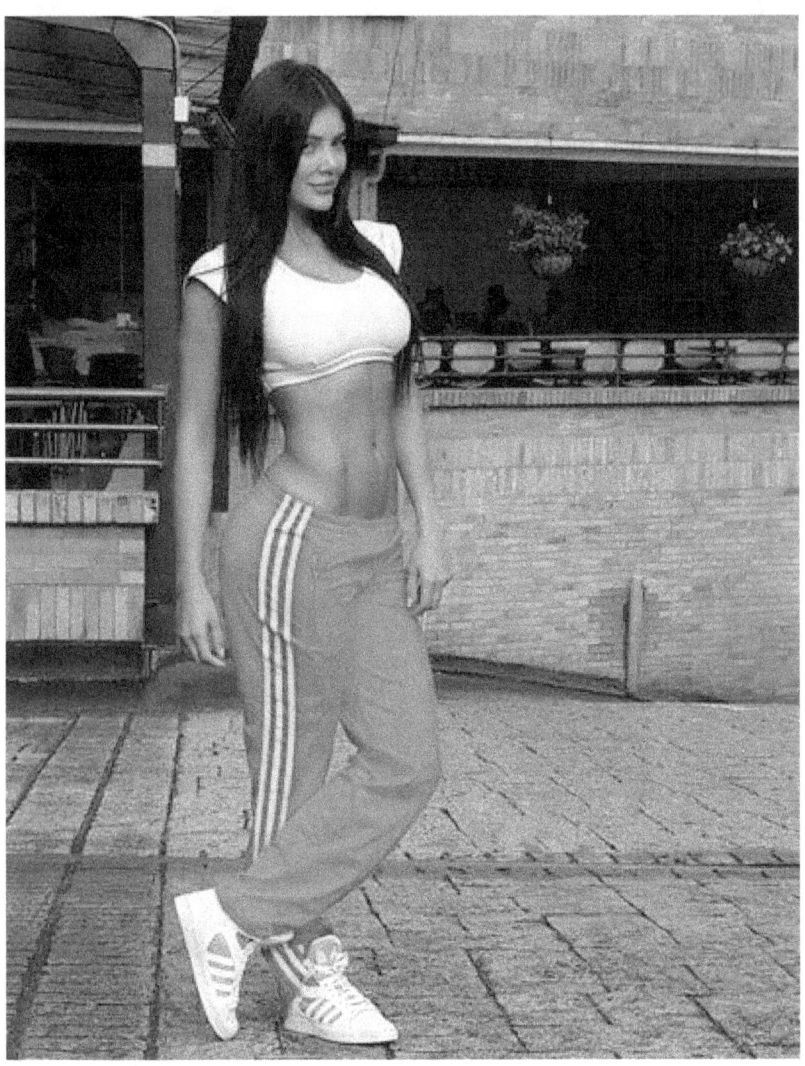

The one month fitness program

Yes it is possible to ramp up your fitness in just a month that's 4 weeks. Yes 4 weeks is all you need to improve your fitness level and physique

The usual fitness programs that you would come across is a 3 month schedule or a 6 months schedule. They can be seen plenty in fitness magazines, but a great physique is possible in just under one month. It doesn't necessarily take toiling for months together to get your feet wet in the gym. Once you completed the hard battle of the first one month, you will notice fitness is within your grasp and working out will come easy to you.

This is more or less an accelerated guideline to a great body and even better fitness. The regime will definitely be demanding but progressive and amazingly beneficial. You will soon be graduating from the basics to high intensity exercises. A month will be enough to build the required muscles and as an added bonus, a toned body to show off.

This routine can be tried out by everyone. You may be just a beginner who doesn't know anything about fitness or who was demotivated by his last attempt to work out. This will get you on the right track in just a short span of one month.

1st week

The program begins with a full body split training. This will make sure you train all major body parts. The three days of the week will be dedicated to performing one exercise for each body part. There should be a gap of one day, on all alternate days. So you are working out essentially for 3 days in a week overall. The exercises are a collection of basic styles, which equally benefit beginners and seasoned body builders. The routine is a mix of free weight movements and work out on machines. These basic moves will help you gain in the long term process.

You will need to work on three sets of each exercise which will ultimately add up to 9 sets in the entire week. Per set will demand 10-12 reps, this doesn't include ab crunches. These sets have been devised to gain muscle size. While starting off with each set, begin with 8 and gradually move to 12 reps. This phenomenon is also called the backwards pyramid or the reverse pyramid count.

Muscle group	Exercise	Sets	Reps
Chest	Bench Press on inclined surface	5	10
Chest	Dumbbell bench press	5	8,8,10,10,12
Chest	Dumbbell fly	5	8,8,10,10,12
Triceps	Rope press down	4	10,10,12,12
Triceps	Dumbbell kickback	3	10
Triceps	Barbell extension	3	10
Calves	Standing Calf lifting	3	25
Calves	Seated Calf lifting	3	25

2nd week

Compared to 1st week, where you trained for just 3 days, you will start working out for 4 days this week. So you will be working on Monday, Tuesday, Thursday and Friday. Wednesday and the Sat- Sun is off for rest. This week will again include split training. First two that's Monday and Tuesday, you will focus on the upper body parts while Thursday and Friday is for lower parts of the body.

A lot of exercises are common between the two weeks, except that an extra move has been added to every exercise. So you are training your muscles but from a different angle. Chest exercise are also of two kinds, both with dumbbells. They together will target your shoulder and elbow joints.

Reverse pyramid phenomenon will apply again here. Ramp up your reps starting from 12 to 15 gradually. This workout will add stamina and muscle endurance.

Muscle group	Exercise	Sets	Reps
Quads	Barbell squats	5	10
Quads	Leg Press	5	8,8,10,10,12
Quads	Leg extension	5	8,8,10,10,12
Hamstrings	Leg curl	3	8,10,12,
Hamstrings	Romanian dead lift	3	8,10,12,
Hamstrings	Leg curl while seated	3	8,10,12,
Abs	Reverse crunch	2	20
Abs	crunch	2	20

3rd week

We continue with training splits in the third week also. You will be going to the gym 6 days in the entire week. You will be working out your shoulders, chest and triceps on the first day. Train your abs and biceps plus your back on the next day. Target the lower body on the third day. This mean focusing on hamstrings, calves and quad muscles. An extra move is added to each routine, keeping in with the trend. The idea is to target your muscles from multiple angles. Each muscle group will be your target with two exercises dedicated to each with 3-4 sets in each exercise. The resultant 16 sets for the bigger body parts and 12 for small ones in the entire week will add a substantial boost to your foundation.

Muscle group	Exercise	Sets	Reps
Shoulders	Dumbbell Overhead press	4	12
Shoulders	Smith machine upright row	3	8,10,12
Shoulders	Dumbbell lateral lift	3	10
Calves	Calf lift while seated	10	10

4th week

This is the final week and is all about turning up the tempo to the maximum. You will train all of four days in the week and the routine is the usual split training. You need to target every part of body one time (abs and calf muscles exercise to train twice). Triceps and chest exercises are paired up, back exercises with biceps and hamstrings with quads. Shoulders gets trained in the process automatically. No surprises or new routines in the final week.

The number of sets are increased up to 5 per move for bigger parts of the body whilst smaller ones get 10 sets. The extra sets ensure that muscles get enough exercise so that you continue your work- out routine easily enough beyond the first month

Muscle group	Exercise	Sets	Reps
Back	Barbell bent over row	5	12
Back	Lat pull down	5	8,8,10,10,12
Back	One arm dumbbell row	5	8,8,8,10,10
Biceps	Barbell curl	4	10,10,12,12
Biceps	Dumbbell curl on inclined surface	3	10
Biceps	Preacher curl machine	3	10
Abs	Crunch	3	20

Please ensure that you stick to the routine laid out above for maximum results and benefit.

Please check out my book series "HOW TO GET ABS" and get in the best shape of your life:

http://www.amazon.com/dp/B00SSFWCPA

http://www.amazon.com/dp/B00QJJFS1C

http://www.amazon.com/dp/B00SX58DUI

Check out my other weight loss and Nutrition Books at:

http://www.amazon.com/dp/B00QH7DY4Y

http://www.amazon.com/dp/B00RVX3KY2

http://www.amazon.com/dp/B00QDHXN7Q

http://www.amazon.com/dp/B00PP8OZJ4

http://www.amazon.com/dp/B00PO0IQIO

You can get access my Free Weight Loss Video at www.achieveitforyou.com

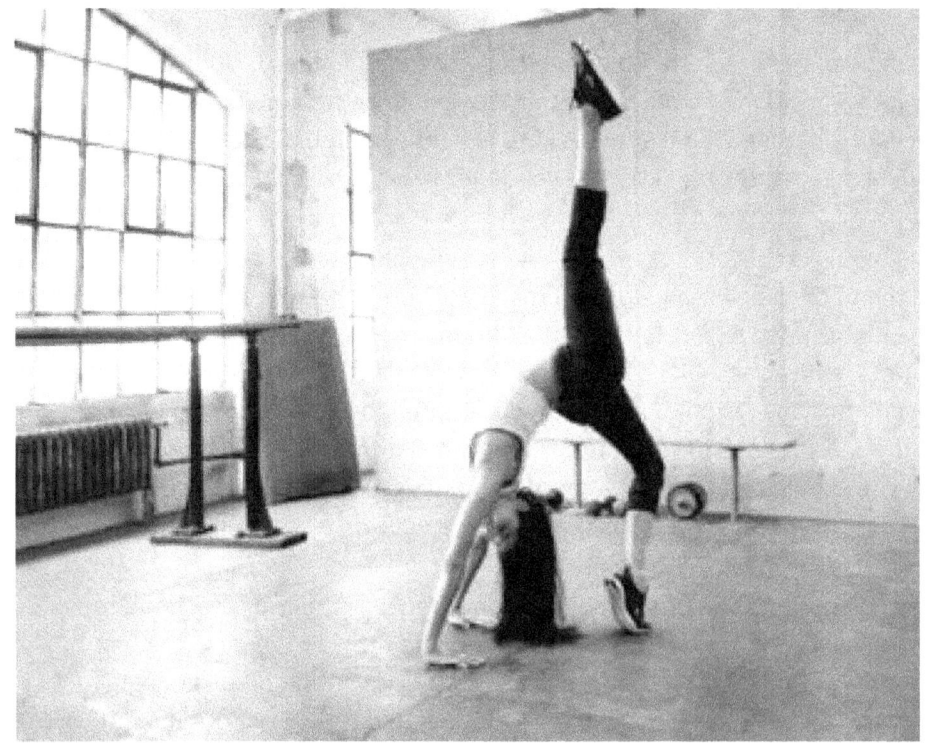

Ab ball exercises

There are various kind of ab exercises out there. The most popular one these days are done with the help of an ab exercise ball. The balls may look harmless but can promise you killer curves in practically no time. The beauty of these exercise balls is that lets the ab muscles to extend beyond 180 degrees, adding to a range of motion which ultimately maximizes the stretch limit. All this would lead to ab contraction and pushes the core into a stage of shock. It also reduces strain on neck and back and move the strain on to your center of the body, which will soon be replaced by the 6 pack ab muscles.

Please follow the below core exercises which are an all-time favorite of fitness enthusiasts. It's important that you include these exercises into your daily ab exercise regime for a comprehensive workout. The exercises will ensure effects from multiple angles which will benefit your lower abs, upper abs, back and oblique. The ball exercise can be done pretty quickly

Ball Ab Crunch

Keep your lower back firm against the top part of the exercise ball. Place your hands behind the head loosely. Lean backwards beyond 180 degrees angle and crunch back upwards. Hold the contraction for second and they start again. Take the process slow to avoid slipping and hurting yourself. The movement should be deliberate and slow with your back touching the ball at all times. When you gain little more proficiency in this exercise and your abs get stronger, you can add to your difficulty level. Hold a dumbbell behind your head and also increase the no of reps.

Ball Jack Knife

Place your feet on the top section of the ball with the upper body extended forward. Understand that you are on all your four. Get into a position of a push up. Your abs should be tightened and upper body steady. Pull the ball towards yourself using your lower abs. The lower back should be straight throughout this routine. You have to constantly resist the tendency to cave in.

Ball Plank

Place your feet again on the top of the ball. Facing downwards, place your forearms on the floor and your legs should be straight and extended all out to the ball. Your upper arms should be below your shoulders. Next, contract your core muscles while balancing the ball in place. Hold this position for 60 seconds, try not to topple over. Your body should be stretched out through the entire routine, don't slump or bend at any point. If you can't hold 60 seconds, try for a smaller time frame and then move up as you practice more. Ideally you should be able to hold position for 1-2 minutes at a stretch.

Ball Roll out

Kneel on your knees with arms placed on the exercise balls. Make sure your forearms reach the top of the ball. Maintain a tight core while keeping your lower back strong and firm. Slowly push the ball forward by rolling it slowly. Keep rolling forward till your abs allow. Your torso should be at angle of 45 degrees to the floor. Hold this position for 5 seconds and then gradually contract your abs and pull back to reach the start position. Repeat 20 times to complete one full set. You can increase the difficultly level by moving your legs to a push up position.

Ball Oblique Crunch

Place your lower back on the exercise ball and settle your body firmly on it. Don't slip off and hurt yourself. Place your hands at the back of your neck and interlink them. Tighten your core, specifically the oblique and very slowly bend forward. Make sure your right elbow points straight at your opposite left knee. Hold the position for one second and return to original position. Relax and repeat the same move with the opposite elbow and knees. Complete 12 reps to make one whole set. Add to the difficulty level by holding a dumbbell in your hands.

Ball Hip elevate

Lie on the floor facing the ceiling. With your back resting on the floor, place your feet on the top of the ball. You heels should be perched firmly on top of the exercise ball so your legs don't slip. Pushing your heels in to the ball, lift your pelvis upwards until your body makes an arch like a bridge. You should be at a 30 degrees angle now. Moving on, tighten your core muscles and straighten your lower back and roll the exercise ball inwards, toward your body. Uplift your torso to make an angle of 75 degrees. Next, bend your knees and push it upwards and hold for a second. Then slowly return to your original position. The getting back to the flat bridge position should be gradual.

Ball back extension

Place your stomach on the ball while facing downwards. You should have placed your exercise ball close to a wall for leg support. The feet should be pressing against the wall. Your body should be as flat as possible and totally stretched out. Now contract your core muscles and lift your torso off the exercise ball. You can take support from your pelvis area. The pelvis should be in contact with the exercise ball at all times. Hold the position for one second and then release to return to start position. Do 20 reps to complete a full set. You can ramp up the difficulty by holding a dumbbell or weights in your hands.

Ball pike

Facing the floor, place your feet on the exercise ball. The toes should be digging into the ball for extra support. Create your balance to make sure the ball doesn't roll out under you. Extend your body to a push up position and contract your core muscles. Start pushing the ball inwards with the help of your feet, especially the toes and raising your torso and back at the same time, keep lifting your torso till you reach a perfect V. Hold the position for 5 seconds and lower down after that and roll back the ball into start position. Repeat 10 times and see best results.

Please check out my book series "HOW TO GET ABS" and get in the best shape of your life:

http://www.amazon.com/dp/B00SSFWCPA

http://www.amazon.com/dp/B00QJJFS1C

http://www.amazon.com/dp/B00SX58DUI

Check out my other weight loss and Nutrition Books at:

http://www.amazon.com/dp/B00QH7DY4Y

http://www.amazon.com/dp/B00RVX3KY2

http://www.amazon.com/dp/B00QDHXN7Q

http://www.amazon.com/dp/B00PP8OZJ4

http://www.amazon.com/dp/B00PO0IQIO

You can get access my Free Weight Loss Video at www.achieveitforyou.com

Why you should hire a personal trainer?

Who are personal trainers? They are fitness professionals who create customized fitness programs to attain your health related goals. Going with a trainer may look tempting because it's a more cost effective option, but is it really effective? Is your personal experience and knowledge enough to help you peak you best, fitness wise.

We can certainly look at some advantages that an experienced trainer brings to the table

Motivation

While working out it can get monotonous really fast. The dropout rates are the highest in gymnasiums. Having a personal trainer by you would definitely help. They will push you to be consistent and keep you from being over frenzied at the same time. Certified trainers can create a foundation and accountability to help develop a style of living which is healthy.

Focused goals

If you have a specific program in mind like a marathon you want to run in or counter your weak heart problems, then getting a trainer will reap good benefits. Focused area of work will require specialized knowledge and professional trainers can help. They will work with you to plan an efficient and safe program which will keep your needs and stamina in mind.

Efficiency

Your trainer will know through experience that routines which are realistic are the best ones. They maximized efficiency and reduce chances of failure. They will help you concentrate on long term results rather than fretting about how much you last today or will tomorrow. He/she will have a schedule charted out for you which will help you reach the maximum result in the shortest span of time.

Improve technique

Suppose you are involved with an extra activity like swimming or cycling, the trainer will provide extra knowledge how the workout schedule can be built around this activity. This maximize the benefit you reap from your workout sessions. The trainer will also tell you what the right form, stand and posture to hold while working out. He/she will also show techniques while working out to improve your stamina and strength. This will add to your mental endurance as well.

You are a beginner

Hiring a personal trainer makes the most sense for beginners. A good fitness trainer will introduce you to techniques which are simple, good and effective. The trainer will pump you with enough motivation and confidence to see you through the entire routine.

New routine

Even if you are a regular at the gym and fairly familiar with all the dos and don'ts and the usual pitfalls, it may sometimes be a good idea to hire a trainer to break through plateaus. You may be in good shape but stuck in the same routine for years without any major difference. This is where the personal trainer will step in to help you break out of the rut. The trainer will not only give a kick to your motivation level but provide you with a brand new routine to break the monotony.

Learn the ropes

You may have been working out for years and yet don't know the nitty gritty of it. You want to design your own routine but understand very little of which body part to work how many days in a week, which food item to avoid and what clothes work best for a work out. A good trainer will help you touch base with the fundamentals and then you carry forward from there.

Prevent injuries

Work out injuries can be tough. Besides discouraging you, it may leave you in a lot of pain and discomfort. A personal trainer will help you maintain the balance and form while you exercise. This ensure you don't stretch or bend wrong and pull a muscle or tear a ligament in the run. The trainer will provide an honest outlook on your strength and endurance, so you know how much you can push yourself and what are your threshold limits.

Lose weight

A common problem that a lot of regular gym goers and fitness enthusiasts face is that the weight loss is extremely slow, practically at snail's pace. This adds to disappointment and finally dropping out. However, if you have resolved to lose weight and get into shape then there should be no stopping you. A personal trainer will be your best option when nothing else is working out. He/she can zero in on why the effectiveness and suggest a more effective replacement.

Spending too much time on machines

You have hit a phase where some machines or routines have become your favorite. This maybe because they come easy to you or you get quick benefits. It is essential to understand that working out should be for a wholesome growth. Just lifting weight or just doing cargo will stunt your fitness levels in the long run. A trainer will be able to guide you better, by keeping you aware of your final goals and prevent getting distracted by your favorite machine

Faster results

Personal trainers will ensure you stick to your regime that have been charted out for you personally. Consistency and hard work will show with time and the results will start pouring in by itself.

There are some ideas to be adhered to while hiring a personal trainer

Their certification or qualification- A certified personal trainer will have a degree in physiology, athletic training, kinesiology and health strengthening. They should also have knowledge of first aid techniques and preferably a CPR certification as well. The certification should come from a recognized university or a reputed organization.

The personal trainer must also possess a documented policy describing services, cost, contract period, and emergency procedures. A medical form clearing all the right boxes should be in place too

Last but definitely not the least is your rapport or comfort level that you will share with your trainer. You should be able to communicate openly and not get pressurized or intimidated by his/her instructions. Any lack of communication may prove fatal leading to injuries.

Please check out my book series "HOW TO GET ABS" and get in the best shape of your life:

http://www.amazon.com/dp/B00SSFWCPA

http://www.amazon.com/dp/B00QJJFS1C

http://www.amazon.com/dp/B00SX58DUI

Check out my other weight loss and Nutrition Books at:

http://www.amazon.com/dp/B00QH7DY4Y

http://www.amazon.com/dp/B00RVX3KY2

http://www.amazon.com/dp/B00QDHXN7Q

http://www.amazon.com/dp/B00PP8OZJ4

http://www.amazon.com/dp/B00PO0IQIO

You can get access my Free Weight Loss Video at www.achieveitforyou.com